I0767887

JUICING

FOR

PROSTATE CANCER

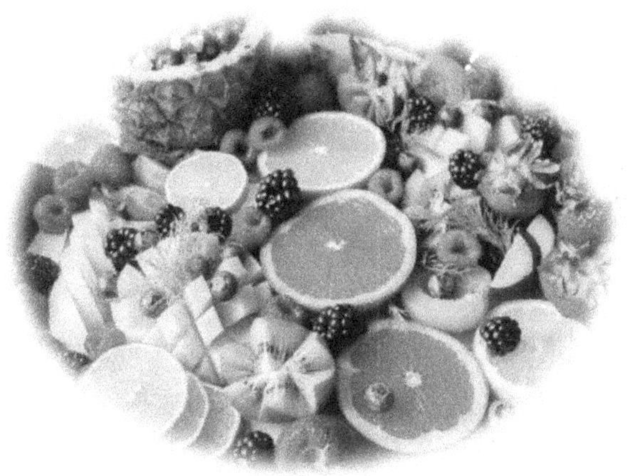

30 NOURISHING AND NUTRIENT-RICH ANTI-INFLAMMATORY HOMEMADE JUICE BLENDS FOR PROSTATE CANCER RECOVERY

Dr. Linda B. Allen

Copyright©2024 by Dr. Linda B. Allen

All rights reserved. No part of this book may be

reproduced, distributed, or transmitted in any form or by

any means, including photocopying, recording, or other

Electronic or mechanical methods, without the prior written

permission of the author, except in the case of brief

Quotations embodied in critical reviews and certain other

Non-commercial uses permitted by copyright law. For

Permission requests, write to the author, addressed

"Attention: Permissions Coordinator,"

dr.lindahelp@gmail.com

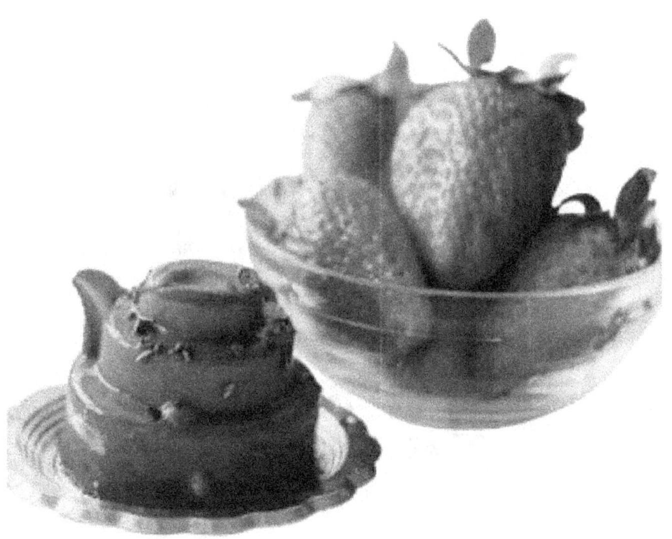

SCAN THE QR-CODE BELOW FOR MORE BOOKS FROM THIS AUTHOR

TABLE OF CONTENTS

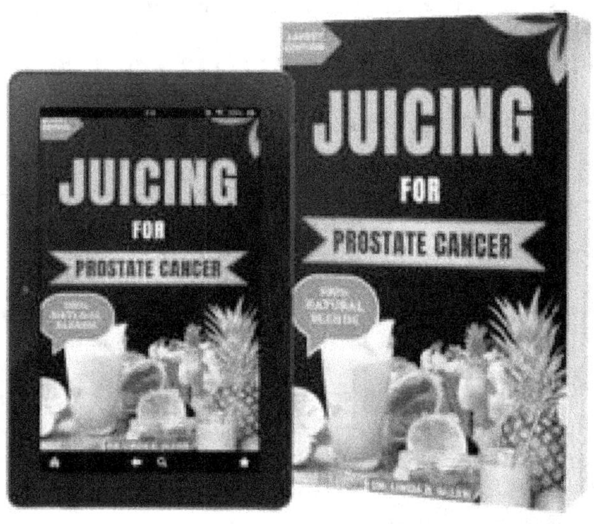

JUICING
FOR
PROSTATE CANCER
JUICING
FOR
PROSTATE CANCER

INTRODUCTION

Greetings, dear reader,

Allow me to extend a warm welcome to the pages of "Juicing for Prostate Cancer: 30 Nourishing and Nutrient-Rich Anti-Inflammatory Homemade Juice Blends for Prostate Cancer Recovery." I am Dr. Linda B. Allen, a seasoned nutrition and diet expert, dedicated to empowering individuals on their journey to optimal health. Throughout my career, I have witnessed the transformative impact of mindful nutrition, and it is with great enthusiasm that I share my insights in this comprehensive guide.

In the following chapters, we will delve into the intricacies of prostate cancer, a condition that affects countless lives. Understanding its nuances, from its origins to potential symptoms, is paramount in navigating the path to recovery. This book aims to serve as a beacon of knowledge, offering not only a profound comprehension of prostate cancer but also practical strategies for its prevention and management.

As a fervent advocate for the healing power of nutrition, I will impart invaluable tips and tricks specific to juicing for prostate cancer. From selecting the right equipment to curating a selection of nutrient-rich ingredients, I aim to guide you through the art of crafting homemade juices that are both delicious and healthful.

Embark with me on a journey through 30 nourishing juice blend recipes and smoothie concoctions, each carefully designed to support prostate cancer recovery. Together, we will explore the harmonious fusion of flavors and nutrients that can contribute to an anti-inflammatory, nutrient-rich approach to health.

Whether you are seeking preventive measures, exploring a complementary approach to conventional treatments, or simply embracing a wellness-focused lifestyle, "Juicing for Prostate Cancer" invites you to unlock the potential of nutrition in your healing journey. Let's navigate these pages together and embark on a path towards vitality, well-being, and prostate health.

Yours in health,

Dr. Linda B. Allen

PART 1

UNDERSTANDING PROSTATE CANCER

Prostate cancer is a significant health concern affecting men worldwide. To navigate this intricate landscape, let's delve into a comprehensive understanding of prostate cancer, covering its nature, potential causes, common signs and symptoms, and practical preventive measures.

What is Prostate Cancer?

Prostate cancer is a type of cancer that originates in the prostate gland, a crucial part of the male reproductive system. The prostate, located just below the bladder, surrounds the urethra and contributes to seminal fluid production. When cells within the prostate undergo abnormal growth, they can form tumors, potentially leading to the development of prostate cancer.

Causes of Prostate Cancer

While the exact cause of prostate cancer remains elusive, several factors contribute to its development. Understanding these potential causes is essential for adopting a proactive approach to one's health.

Common contributors include:

Age: Prostate cancer risk rises with age, especially after the age of fifty.

Genetics and Family History: Individuals with a family history of prostate cancer, especially if a close relative has been affected, may have an increased risk.

Race and Ethnicity: African American men have a higher incidence of prostate cancer, emphasizing the role of genetics and ethnicity in susceptibility.

Lifestyle Factors: Dietary choices, exposure to certain environmental elements, and lifestyle habits can influence the likelihSood of developing prostate cancer.

Hormonal Factors: Changes in hormonal balance, particularly an increase in levels of male hormones like testosterone, may contribute to the development of prostate cancer.

Signs and Symptoms of Prostate Cancer

Recognizing the signs and symptoms of prostate cancer is crucial for early detection and intervention. While early-stage prostate cancer may be asymptomatic, the following indicators may arise as the disease progresses:

Urinary Changes: Increased frequency of urination, difficulty initiating or stopping urine flow, and blood in the urine may be signs of prostate cancer.

Pelvic Discomfort: Pain or discomfort in the pelvic area, lower back, or thighs may be indicative of advanced prostate cancer.

Erectile Dysfunction: Prostate cancer is a possible cause of erectile dysfunction, while it can also be brought on by a number of other conditions.

Preventive Measures for Prostate Cancer

Proactive measures can significantly reduce the risk of developing prostate cancer.

Here are practical steps for maintaining prostate health:

Healthy Diet: Adopt a diet high in fruit, vegetables, whole grains, and balance. Include sources of omega-3 fatty acids, like fatty fish and flaxseeds.

Regular Exercise: Engage in regular physical activity to promote overall health and reduce the risk of prostate cancer.

Screening and Early Detection: Discuss with your healthcare provider about appropriate screening methods, such as prostate-specific antigen (PSA) tests and digital rectal exams, especially if you have risk factors.

Maintain a Healthy Weight: Obesity has been linked to an increased risk of prostate cancer, making weight management an essential aspect of preventive care.

Limit Red Meat and High-Fat Dairy: While the evidence is not conclusive, some studies suggest that reducing the intake of red meat and high-fat dairy products may contribute to a lower risk of prostate cancer.

TIPS AND TRICKS FOR OPTIMAL HEALTH

As we embark on the journey of juicing for prostate cancer, it's essential to explore the nuanced tips and tricks that can enhance not only the flavor of your juices but also their potential health benefits. From selecting the right juicing equipment to choosing the most beneficial ingredients and ensuring proper storage, each step is a crucial component of your path to wellness.

Choosing the Right Juicing Equipment

Investing in the right juicing equipment is the foundation for a successful juicing journey. Here are some pointers to help you choose:

Masticating Juicers: Opt for masticating juicers, also known as slow juicers, as they operate at lower speeds, minimizing heat buildup and oxidation. This preserves the nutritional integrity of your juice, ensuring maximum health benefits.

Ease of Cleaning: Choose a juicer with parts that are easy to disassemble and clean. This convenience not only saves time but also encourages regular juicing without the hassle of intricate cleaning processes.

Juice Yield: Consider the efficiency of juice extraction. Look for juicers that maximize the yield from your chosen ingredients, ensuring you get the most nutrition from every fruit and vegetable.

Noise Level: If noise is a concern, consider juicers with quieter operation, especially if you plan to incorporate juicing into your daily routine without disturbing the household.

Choosing the Juicing Ingredients

Selecting the right ingredients is pivotal to the effectiveness of juicing for prostate health. Here are guidelines for making optimal choices:

Colorful Variety: Embrace a diverse array of fruits and vegetables with vibrant colors. Different colors signify various phytonutrients, each contributing to overall health.

Cruciferous Vegetables: Include cruciferous vegetables like broccoli, kale, and cabbage, known for their anti-cancer properties. These vegetables contain compounds that may have protective effects against prostate cancer.

Berries: Berries, rich in antioxidants, can play a crucial role in reducing inflammation. Consider incorporating blueberries, strawberries, and raspberries into your juice blends.

Turmeric and Ginger: Both turmeric and ginger have potent anti-inflammatory properties. Adding a small amount to your juices can contribute not only to flavor but also to the potential health benefits.

Leafy Greens: Include leafy greens such as spinach and kale for their wealth of vitamins, minerals, and antioxidants. These greens can be powerful allies in supporting overall health.

How to Perfectly Store Your Juice

Preserving the freshness and nutritional content of your juices is key to maximizing their benefits. Follow these storage tips:

Air-Tight Containers: Store your juice in air-tight containers to minimize exposure to oxygen, which can lead to oxidation and nutrient degradation.

Refrigeration: Immediately refrigerate your juice after preparation to slow down the enzymatic reactions that can occur at room temperature.

Dark Containers: Choose dark containers to protect your juice from light exposure, which can also contribute to nutrient loss.

Minimal Airspace: When storing juice, minimize the airspace in the container to reduce oxidation. Consider using smaller containers to match your serving size.

Consume Promptly: While freshly prepared juice is ideal, if you need to store it, consume it within 24 to 48 hours to ensure maximum freshness and nutritional value.

PART 3

NOURISHING JUICE BLEND RECIPES

1. Prostate Protector Green Blend

Ingredients:

- 1 cup kale
- 1 cup spinach
- 1 cucumber
- 1 green apple
- 1/2 lemon (peeled)
- 1-inch ginger (peeled)

Preparation:

1. Wash all the ingredients thoroughly.
2. Core the apple and cut it into wedges.
3. Juice all ingredients in a masticating juicer.
4. Stir well and pour into a glass.

Portion Size: 1 serving

Time: 10 minutes

Nutritional Information: Rich in antioxidants, vitamins A and C, and anti-inflammatory properties.

2. Berry Bliss Antioxidant Blend

Ingredients:

- 1 cup blueberries
- 1 cup strawberries
- 1/2 cup raspberries
- 1 beet (peeled)
- 1 orange (peeled)

Preparation:

1. Wash berries and peel the orange.
2. Cut the beet into smaller chunks.
3. Juice all ingredients together.
4. Mix well and serve over ice.

Portion Size: 1 serving

Time: 10 minutes

Nutritional Information: High in antioxidants, vitamin C, and anti-inflammatory compounds.

3. Turmeric Twist Healing Blend

Ingredients:

- 2 carrots
- 1 orange (peeled)
- 1/2-inch turmeric root (peeled)
- 1/2-inch ginger (peeled)
- 1 apple

Preparation:

1. Wash all the ingredients.
2. Cut the carrots and apple into smaller pieces.
3. Juice all ingredients using a masticating juicer.
4. Stir well and serve.

Portion Size: 1 serving

Time: 15 minutes

Nutritional Information: Anti-inflammatory, rich in vitamin A and C, and provides the benefits of turmeric.

4. Prostate Power Citrus Blend

Ingredients:

- 2 grapefruits (peeled)
- 2 oranges (peeled)
- 1 lemon (peeled)
- 1/2-inch ginger (peeled)

Preparation:

1. Peel the citrus fruits.
2. Cut them into smaller segments.
3. Juice all ingredients.
4. Mix well and enjoy.

Portion Size: 1 serving

Time: 10 minutes

Nutritional Information: High in vitamin C, antioxidants, and anti-inflammatory properties.

5. Green Goddess Detox Blend

Ingredients:

- 1 cup kale
- 1 cup cucumber
- 1 celery stalk
- 1 green apple
- 1/2 lemon (peeled)
- 1/2 cup parsley

Preparation:

1. Wash all the ingredients.
2. Core the apple and cut it into wedges.
3. Juice all ingredients together.
4. Stir well and pour into a glass.

Portion Size: 1 serving

Time: 12 minutes

Nutritional Information: Detoxifying, rich in vitamins K and C, and provides a boost of chlorophyll.

6. Pomegranate Powerhouse Blend

Ingredients:

- 1 cup pomegranate seeds
- 1 cup blueberries
- 1 apple
- 1/2 lemon (peeled)
- 1-inch ginger (peeled)

Preparation:

1. Wash all the ingredients.
2. Core the apple and cut it into wedges.
3. Juice all ingredients using a masticating juicer.
4. Mix well and serve over ice.

Portion Size: 1 serving

Time: 10 minutes

Nutritional Information: Rich in antioxidants, vitamin C, and anti-inflammatory compounds.

7. Carrot-Orange Energizer Blend

Ingredients:

- 4 carrots
- 2 oranges (peeled)
- 1/2-inch ginger (peeled)

Preparation:

1. Wash and peel the carrots.
2. Peel the oranges.
3. Cut carrots and oranges into smaller pieces.
4. Juice all ingredients together.
5. Stir well and serve.

Portion Size: 1 serving

Time: 12 minutes

Nutritional Information: High in beta-carotene, vitamin C, and anti-inflammatory properties.

8. Pineapple Paradise Prostate Blend

Ingredients:

- 1 cup pineapple chunks
- 1 cucumber
- 1 green apple
- 1/2 lemon (peeled)
- Mint leaves (optional)

Preparation:

1. Wash all the ingredients.
2. Core the apple and cut it into wedges.
3. Juice all ingredients together.
4. Garnish with mint leaves if desired.

Portion Size: 1 serving

Time: 10 minutes

Nutritional Information: Contains bromelain from pineapple, vitamin C, and anti-inflammatory properties.

9. Beetroot Berry Boost Blend

Ingredients:

- 1 beet (peeled)
- 1 cup mixed berries (blueberries, raspberries, strawberries)
- 1 orange (peeled)
- 1/2-inch ginger (peeled)

Preparation:

1. Wash berries and peel the orange.
2. Cut the beet into smaller chunks.
3. Juice all ingredients together.
4. Mix well and serve.

Portion Size: 1 serving

Time: 12 minutes

Nutritional Information: High in antioxidants, folate, and anti-inflammatory compounds.

10. Mango Tango Prostate Soother Blend

Ingredients:

- 1 cup mango chunks
- 1 cup papaya chunks
- 1/2 cup pineapple chunks
- 1/2 lemon (peeled)
- 1/2-inch turmeric root (peeled)

Preparation:

1. Peel and chop the mango, papaya, and pineapple.
2. Cut the turmeric into smaller pieces.
3. Juice all ingredients together.
4. Stir well and enjoy.

Portion Size: 1 serving

Time: 15 minutes

Nutritional Information: Rich in vitamins A and C, anti-inflammatory, and provides digestive enzymes.

11. Tomato Tango Immune Booster Blend

Ingredients:

- 2 cups tomatoes
- 1 cup red bell pepper
- 1 celery stalk
- 1/2 cup parsley
- 1/2 lemon (peeled)

Preparation:

1. Wash and chop the tomatoes and red bell pepper.
2. Cut the celery into smaller pieces.
3. Juice all ingredients together.
4. Mix well and serve over ice.

Portion Size: 1 serving

Time: 12 minutes

Nutritional Information: Rich in lycopene, vitamin C, and immune-boosting properties.

12. Kiwi-Citrus Vitality Blend

Ingredients:

- 3 kiwis (peeled)
- 2 oranges (peeled)
- 1/2 lemon (peeled)
- 1-inch ginger (peeled)

Preparation:

1. Peel and slice the kiwis.
2. Cut the oranges into wedges.
3. Juice all ingredients using a masticating juicer.
4. Stir well and serve.

Portion Size: 1 serving

Time: 10 minutes

Nutritional Information: High in vitamin C, antioxidants, and digestive enzymes.

13. Spinach Avocado Powerhouse Blend

Ingredients:

- 2 cups spinach
- 1 avocado
- 1 cucumber
- 1/2 lemon (peeled)
- 1/2-inch ginger (peeled)

Preparation:

1. Wash the spinach and peel the lemon.
2. Cut the avocado and cucumber into smaller pieces.
3. Juice all ingredients together.
4. Blend until smooth and enjoy.

Portion Size: 1 serving

Time: 15 minutes

Nutritional Information: Rich in leafy greens, healthy fats, and immune-boosting properties.

14. Cabbage Crunch Detox Blend

Ingredients:

- 1 cup red cabbage
- 1 cup green cabbage
- 1 apple
- 1/2 lemon (peeled)
- 1/2-inch turmeric root (peeled)

Preparation:

1. Wash and shred the red and green cabbage.
2. Core the apple and cut it into wedges.
3. Juice all ingredients using a masticating juicer.
4. Mix well and serve.

Portion Size: 1 serving

Time: 12 minutes

Nutritional Information: Detoxifying, anti-inflammatory, and rich in vitamins and minerals.

15. Broccoli Burst Antioxidant Blend

Ingredients:

- 1 cup broccoli florets
- 1 cup pineapple chunks
- 1/2 lemon (peeled)
- 1/2-inch ginger (peeled)

Preparation:

1. Wash the broccoli and peel the lemon.
2. Cut the broccoli into smaller florets.
3. Juice all ingredients together.
4. Stir well and serve over ice.

Portion Size: 1 serving

Time: 12 minutes

Nutritional Information: High in antioxidants, vitamin C, and anti-inflammatory compounds.

16. Watermelon Wonder Hydration Blend

Ingredients:

- 2 cups watermelon chunks
- 1 cucumber
- 1/2 lemon (peeled)
- Mint leaves (optional)

Preparation:

1. Remove seeds from the watermelon and cut it into chunks.
2. Wash the cucumber and peel the lemon.
3. Juice all ingredients using a masticating juicer.
4. Garnish with mint leaves if desired.

Portion Size: 1 serving

Time: 10 minutes

Nutritional Information: Hydrating, rich in vitamins A and C, and refreshing.

17. Cauliflower Cleanse Detox Blend

Ingredients:

- 1 cup cauliflower florets
- 1 cucumber
- 1 green apple
- 1/2 lemon (peeled)
- 1/2-inch ginger (peeled)

Preparation:

1. Wash the cauliflower and peel the lemon.
2. Cut the cauliflower into smaller florets.
3. Juice all ingredients together.
4. Mix well and serve over ice.

Portion Size: 1 serving

Time: 12 minutes

Nutritional Information: Detoxifying, anti-inflammatory, and rich in vitamins and minerals.

18. Basil Berry Infusion Blend

Ingredients:

- One cup of mixed berries (blueberries, strawberries, raspberries)
- 1/2 cup basil leaves
- 1 cucumber
- 1/2 lemon (peeled)

Preparation:

1. Wash berries, cucumber, and basil leaves.
2. Cut the cucumber into smaller pieces.
3. Juice all ingredients together.
4. Stir well and serve.

Portion Size: 1 serving

Time: 10 minutes

Nutritional Information: High in antioxidants, vitamin C, and provides a refreshing twist.

19. Lemon Lavender Relaxation Blend

Ingredients:

- 2 lemons (peeled)
- 1/2 cup lavender leaves
- 1 cucumber
- 1 green apple

Preparation:

1. Peel the lemons and wash the cucumber.
2. Cut the cucumber and apple into smaller pieces.
3. Juice all ingredients using a masticating juicer.
4. Mix well and serve over ice.

Portion Size: 1 serving

Time: 12 minutes

Nutritional Information: Refreshing, rich in vitamin C, and includes the calming essence of lavender.

20. Almond Joy Prostate Support Blend

Ingredients:

- 1 cup almond milk
- 1 banana
- 2 tablespoons chia seeds
- 1 tablespoon almond butter
- 1/2 teaspoon cinnamon
- 1/2 teaspoon turmeric powder

Preparation:

1. Peel the banana.
2. In a blender, combine all ingredients.
3. Blend until smooth and creamy.
4. Pour into a glass and sprinkle a pinch of cinnamon on top.

Portion Size: 1 serving

Time: 5 minutes

Nutritional Information: Prostate-supportive, rich in omega-3 fatty acids, and provides a satisfying blend of flavors.

1. Berry Blast Prostate Support Smoothie

Ingredients:

- One cup of mixed berries (blueberries, strawberries, raspberries)
- 1/2 cup Greek yogurt
- 1 tablespoon flaxseeds
- 1/2 cup almond milk
- 1 tablespoon honey
- Ice cubes (optional)

Preparation:

1. Wash berries and combine with Greek yogurt, flaxseeds, almond milk, and honey in a blender.
2. Blend until smooth.
3. Add ice cubes if desired and blend again.
4. Pour into a glass and enjoy.

Portion Size: 1 serving

Time: 5 minutes

Nutritional Information: High in antioxidants, omega-3 fatty acids, and probiotics.

2. Green Powerhouse Prostate Smoothie

Ingredients:

- 2 cups spinach
- 1/2 cucumber
- 1/2 avocado
- 1/2 lemon (peeled)
- 1 tablespoon chia seeds
- 1 cup coconut water
- Ice cubes (optional)

Preparation:

1. Wash spinach and peel the cucumber and lemon.
2. Combine spinach, cucumber, avocado, lemon, chia seeds, and coconut water in a blender.
3. Blend until smooth.
4. Add ice cubes if desired and blend again.
5. Pour into a glass and enjoy.

Portion Size: 1 serving

Time: 7 minutes

Nutritional Information: Rich in vitamins A and C, fiber, and healthy fats.

3. Tropical Turmeric Prostate Soothing Smoothie

Ingredients:

- 1 cup pineapple chunks
- 1/2 banana
- 1/2 teaspoon turmeric powder
- 1/2 teaspoon ginger (freshly grated)
- 1 tablespoon hemp seeds
- 1 cup coconut milk
- Ice cubes (optional)

Preparation:

1. Peel the banana and wash pineapple.
2. Combine pineapple, banana, turmeric powder, ginger, hemp seeds, and coconut milk in a blender.
3. Blend until smooth.
4. Add ice cubes if desired and blend again.
5. Pour into a glass and enjoy.

Portion Size: 1 serving

Time: 6 minutes

Nutritional Information: Anti-inflammatory, rich in vitamin C, and provides essential fatty acids.

4. Prostate Defense Blueberry Smoothie

Ingredients:

- 1 cup blueberries
- 1/2 cup Greek yogurt
- 1 tablespoon pumpkin seeds
- 1/2 cup almond milk
- 1 tablespoon honey
- Ice cubes (optional)

Preparation:

1. Wash blueberries and combine with Greek yogurt, pumpkin seeds, almond milk, and honey in a blender.
2. Blend until smooth.
3. Add ice cubes if desired and blend again.
4. Pour into a glass and enjoy.

Portion Size: 1 serving

Time: 5 minutes

Nutritional Information: High in antioxidants, probiotics, and zinc.

5. Papaya Passion Prostate-Boosting Smoothie

Ingredients:

- 1 cup papaya chunks
- 1/2 cup mango chunks
- 1/2 banana
- 1/2 teaspoon turmeric powder
- 1 tablespoon chia seeds
- 1 cup coconut water
- Ice cubes (optional)

Preparation:

1. Peel the banana and wash papaya and mango.
2. Combine papaya, mango, banana, turmeric powder, chia seeds, and coconut water in a blender.
3. Blend until smooth.
4. Add ice cubes if desired and blend again.
5. Pour into a glass and enjoy.

Portion Size: 1 serving

Time: 7 minutes

Nutritional Information: Anti-inflammatory, rich in vitamins A and C, and provides essential fatty acids.

6. Kale and Pineapple Prostate-Care Smoothie

Ingredients:

- 2 cups kale
- 1 cup pineapple chunks
- 1/2 banana
- 1 tablespoon flaxseeds
- 1 cup almond milk
- Ice cubes (optional)

Preparation:

1. Wash kale and peel banana.
2. Combine kale, pineapple, banana, flaxseeds, and almond milk in a blender.
3. Blend until smooth.
4. Add ice cubes if desired and blend again.
5. Pour into a glass and enjoy.

Portion Size: 1 serving

Time: 6 minutes

Nutritional Information: Rich in antioxidants, fiber, and omega-3 fatty acids.

7. Avocado Almond Bliss Prostate Support Smoothie

Ingredients:

- 1/2 avocado
- 1/2 cup spinach
- 1/2 cup blueberries
- 1 tablespoon almond butter
- 1 cup almond milk
- 1 tablespoon honey
- Ice cubes (optional)

Preparation:

1. Peel the avocado and wash spinach.
2. Combine avocado, spinach, blueberries, almond butter, almond milk, and honey in a blender.
3. Blend until smooth.
4. Add ice cubes if desired and blend again.
5. Pour into a glass and enjoy.

Portion Size: 1 serving

Time: 6 minutes

Nutritional Information: Rich in healthy fats, antioxidants, and vitamin E.

8. Prostate Protector Pumpkin Spice Smoothie

Ingredients:

- 1/2 cup pumpkin puree
- 1/2 banana
- 1/2 teaspoon cinnamon
- 1/4 teaspoon nutmeg
- 1 tablespoon chia seeds
- 1 cup coconut milk
- Ice cubes (optional)

Preparation:

1. Peel the banana.
2. Combine pumpkin puree, banana, cinnamon, nutmeg, chia seeds, and coconut milk in a blender.
3. Blend until smooth.
4. Add ice cubes if desired and blend again.
5. Pour into a glass and enjoy.

Portion Size: 1 serving

Time: 5 minutes

Nutritional Information: Rich in fiber, beta-carotene, and omega-3 fatty acids.

9. Strawberry Banana Prostate Care Smoothie

Ingredients:

- 1 cup strawberries
- 1/2 banana
- 1/2 cup Greek yogurt
- 1 tablespoon flaxseeds
- 1 cup almond milk
- 1 tablespoon honey
- Ice cubes (optional)

Preparation:

1. Wash strawberries and peel the banana.
2. Combine strawberries, banana, Greek yogurt, flaxseeds, almond milk, and honey in a blender.
3. Blend until smooth.
4. Add ice cubes if desired and blend again.
5. Pour into a glass and enjoy.

Portion Size: 1 serving

Time: 5 minutes

Nutritional Information: High in antioxidants, probiotics, and omega-3 fatty acids.

10. Coconut Berry Prostate Defense Smoothie

Ingredients:

- One cup of mixed berries (blueberries, strawberries, raspberries)
- 1/2 cup coconut milk
- 1/2 banana
- 1 tablespoon chia seeds
- 1 tablespoon coconut flakes
- Ice cubes (optional)

Preparation:

1. Wash berries and peel the banana.
2. Combine berries, coconut milk, banana, chia seeds, and coconut flakes in a blender.
3. Blend until smooth.
4. Add ice cubes if desired and blend again.
5. Pour into a glass and enjoy.

Portion Size: 1 serving

Time: 5 minutes

Nutritional Information: Rich in antioxidants, fiber, and healthy fats.

CONCLUSION

As we conclude this exploration into the world of juicing and smoothies tailored for prostate health, it is crucial to recognize the transformative power of incorporating these vibrant blends into one's lifestyle.

Through a comprehensive understanding of prostate cancer, we've unveiled the significance of proactive measures, emphasizing the role of nutrition in fostering a resilient foundation. The curated juice blends and smoothie recipes provided in this guide are not mere concoctions; they are crafted with a purpose, to infuse the body with an arsenal of nutrients that may contribute to prostate health and overall well-being.

From the Prostate Protector Green Blend to the comforting Coconut Berry Prostate Defense Smoothie, each recipe carries a unique blend of vitamins, antioxidants, and anti-inflammatory agents. These ingredients, carefully selected for their potential benefits, serve as allies in the quest for optimal health.

Choosing the right juicing equipment, selecting a spectrum of colorful and nutrient-dense ingredients, and storing your creations with care all play pivotal roles in maximizing the efficacy of these healthful concoctions.

Is my sincere hope that this guide serves as a valuable resource, inspiring you to embrace a lifestyle marked by conscious nutritional choices and a commitment to overall well-being.

Remember, the path to recovery and management is unique for each individual. Consultation with healthcare professionals, regular screenings, and a holistic approach to health will continue to be essential components of your wellness journey. As you embark on this path, may the vibrant hues of these juice blends and smoothies reflect the vitality that awaits you on your road to prostate health and beyond.

Here's to nourishing your body, uplifting your spirit, and embracing the journey towards a healthier, more vibrant life.

www.ingramcontent.com/pod-product-compliance
Lightning Source LLC
Chambersburg PA
CBHW070734260726

48660CB00007B/2846